HOW TO HAVE **SEX** IN PUBLIC WITHOUT BEING NOTICED

MARCEL FEIGEL · ILLUSTRATIONS BY BRIAN HEATON

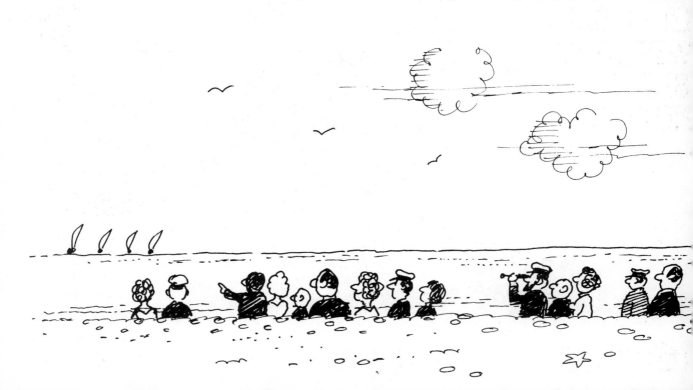

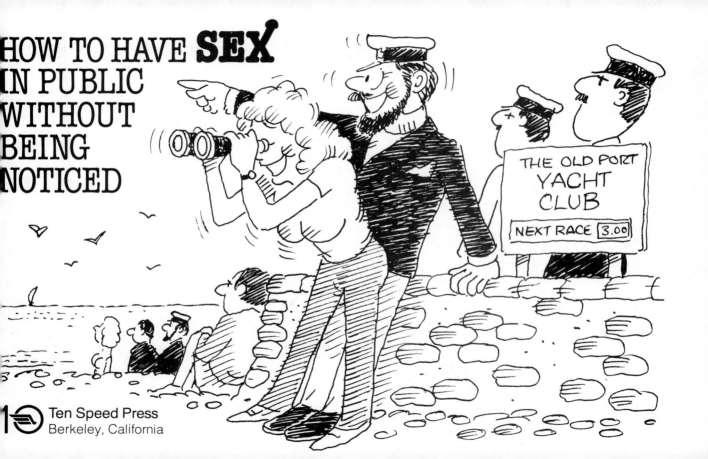

TEN SPEED PRESS
PO Box 7123
Berkeley, California 94707

You may order single copies direct from the publisher for $2.95 + $1.00
for postage and handling (California residents add 6% state sales tax;
Bay Area residents add 6½%).

Library of Congress Catalog Number: 83-50566
ISBN: 0-89815-115-5

Printed in the United States of America

10   9   8   7   6   5   4   3

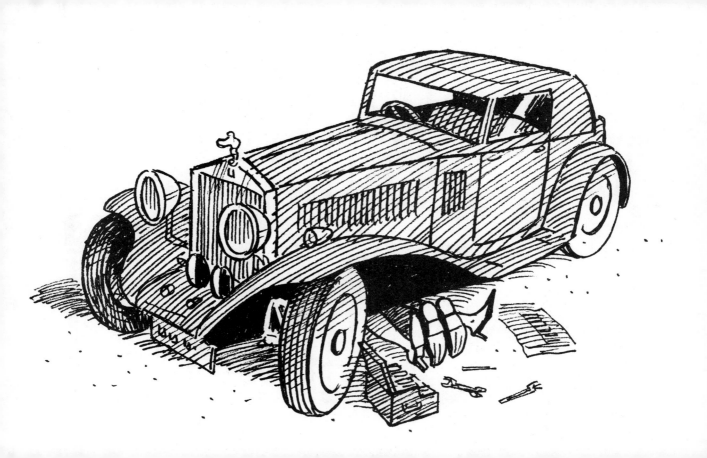

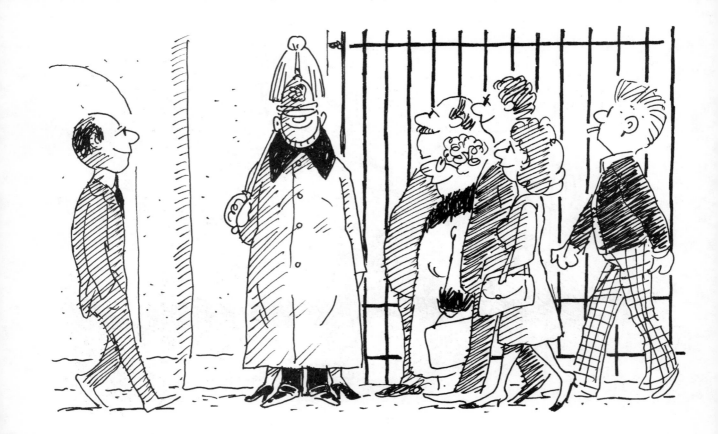

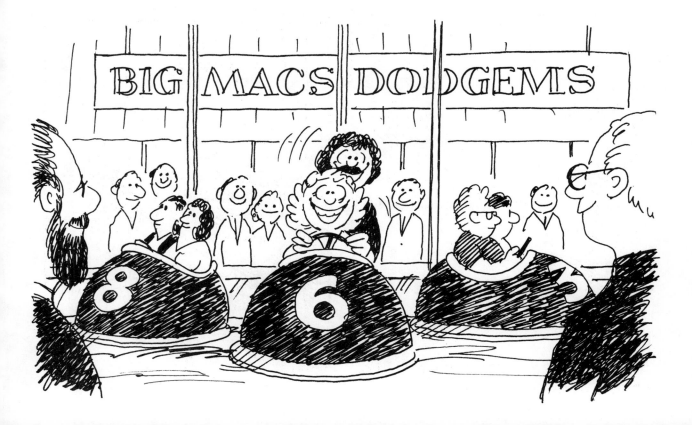

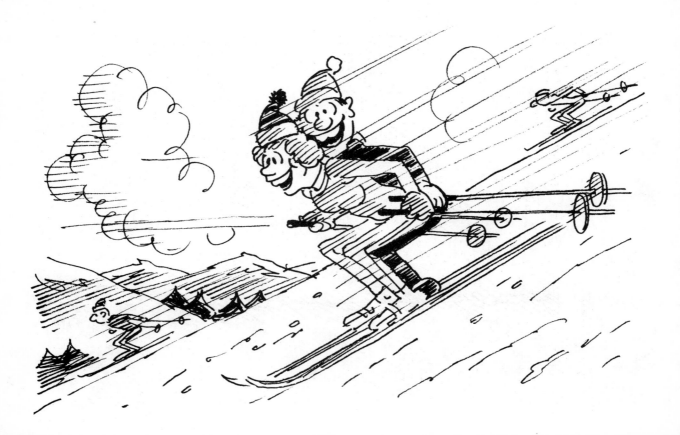

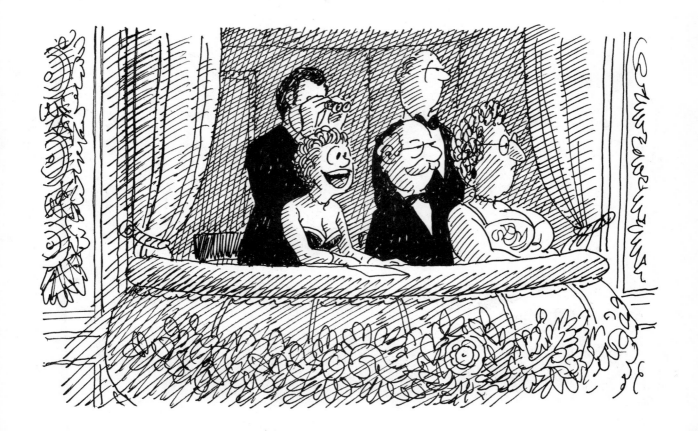

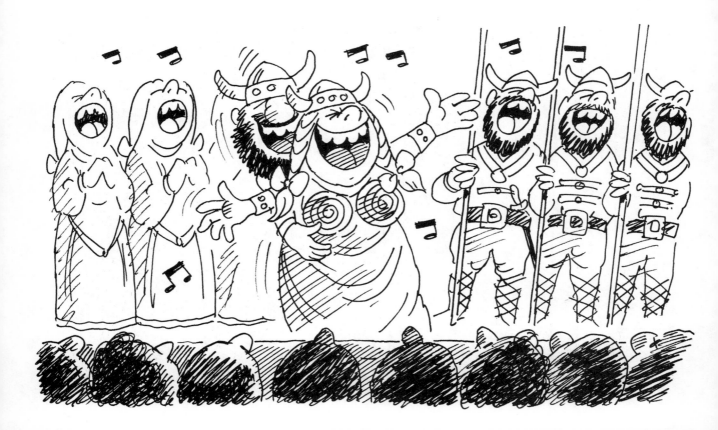

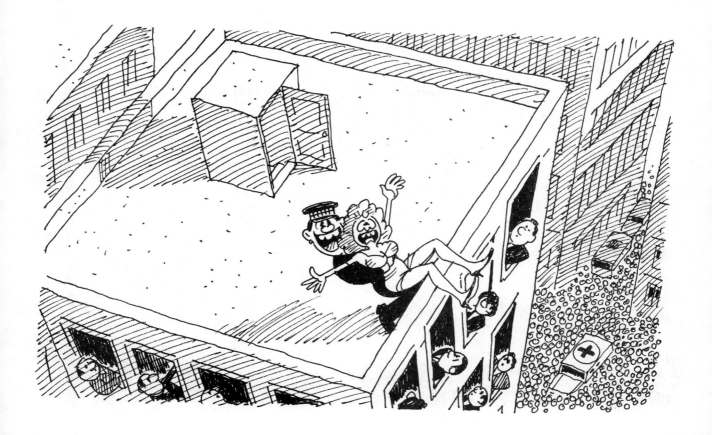

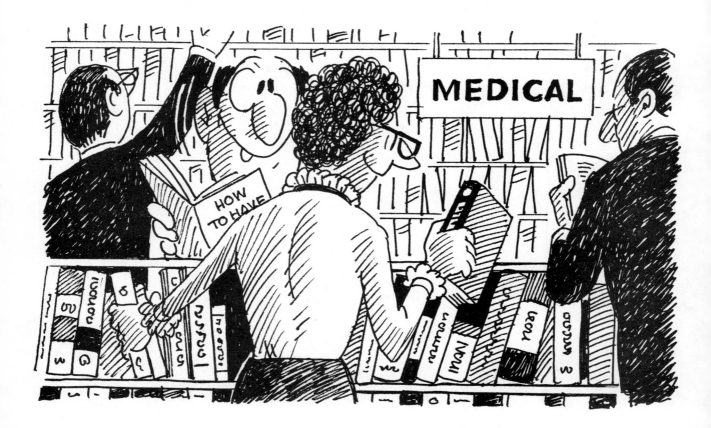

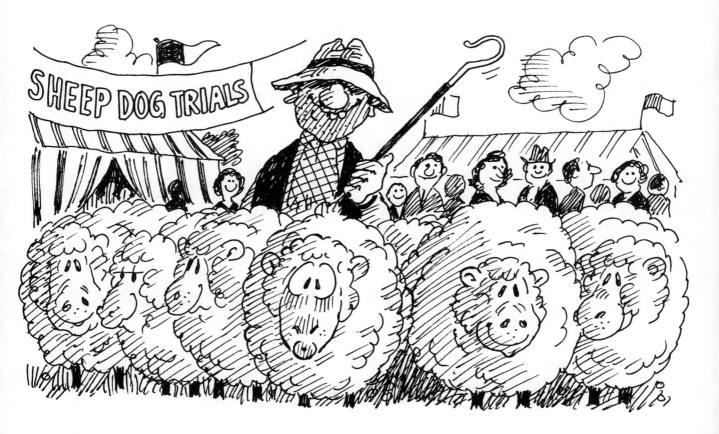

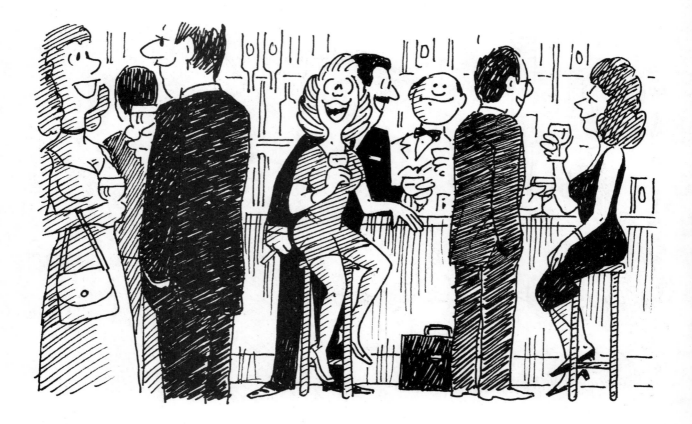

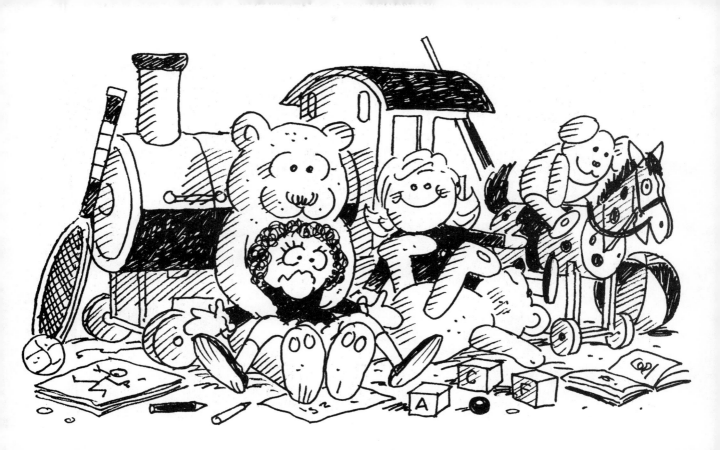

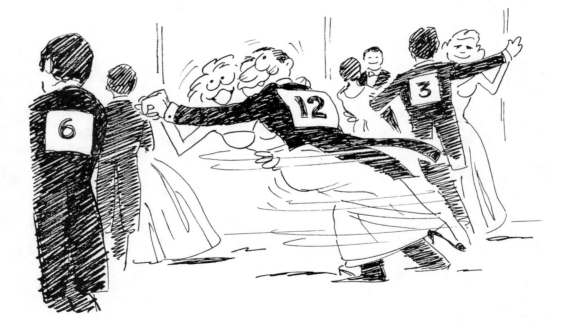

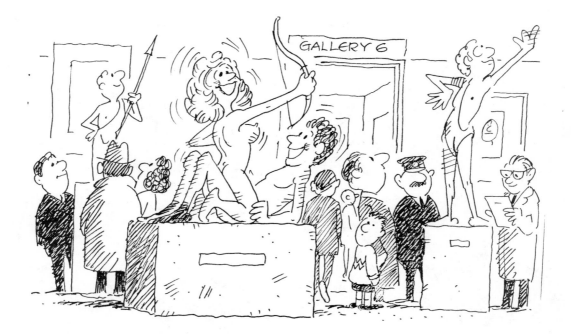

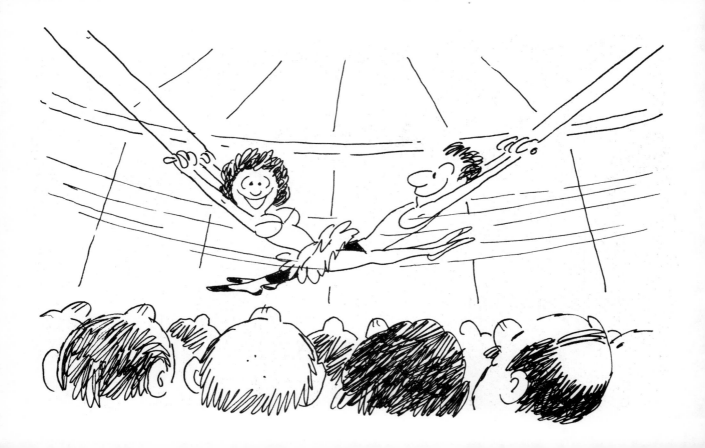

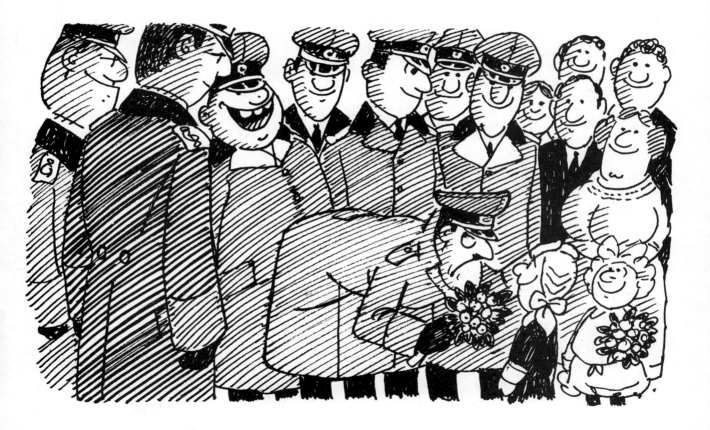

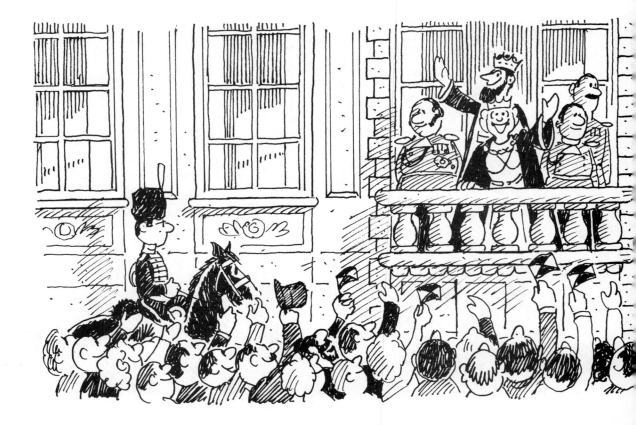

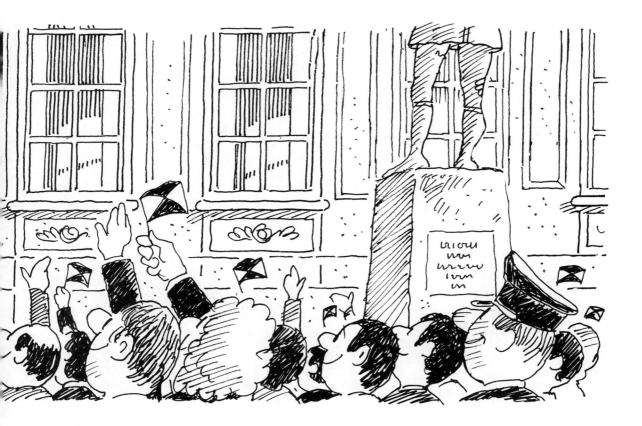

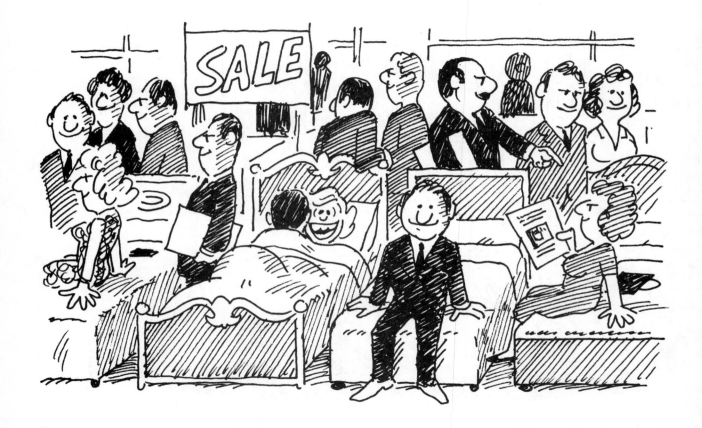

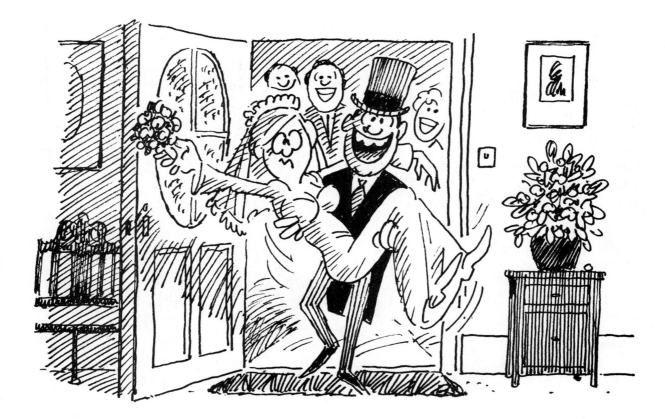

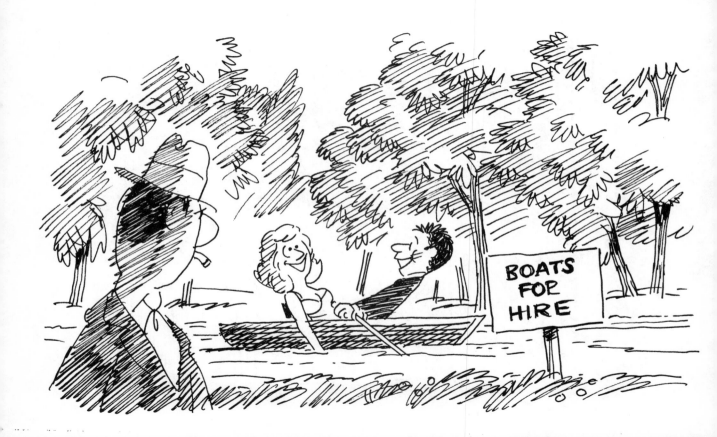

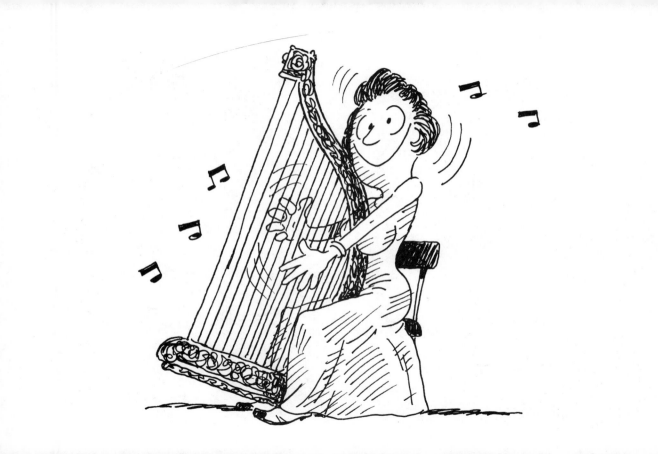

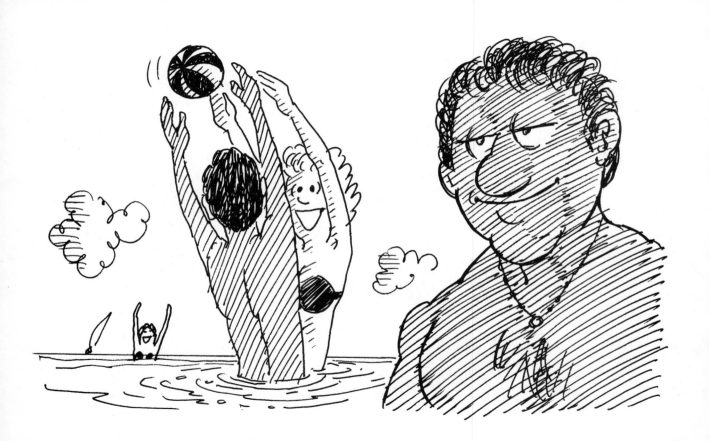

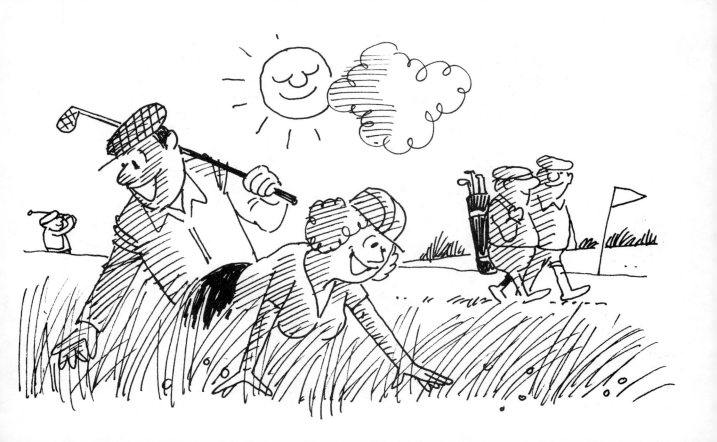

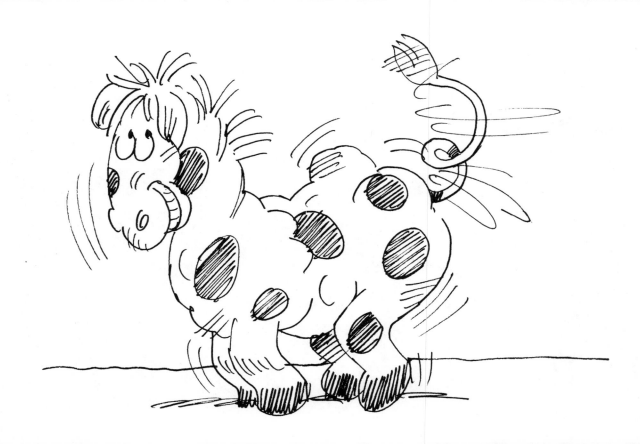

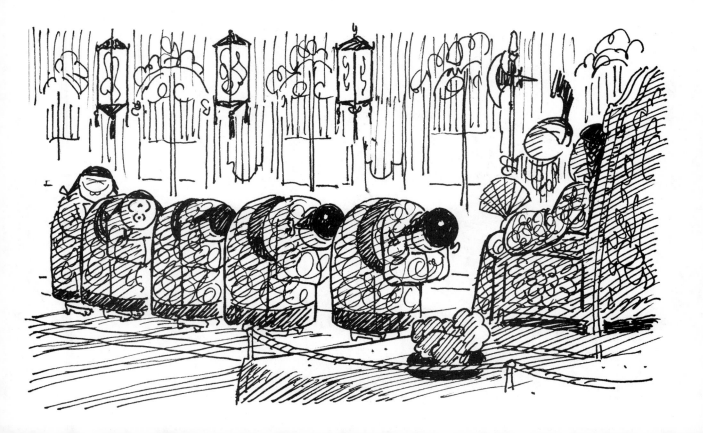

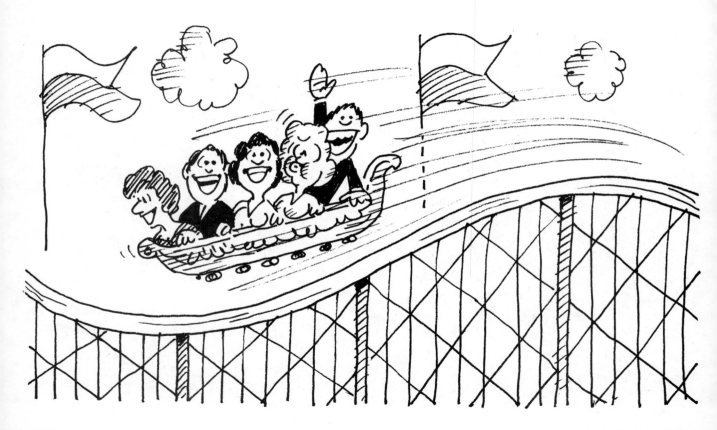

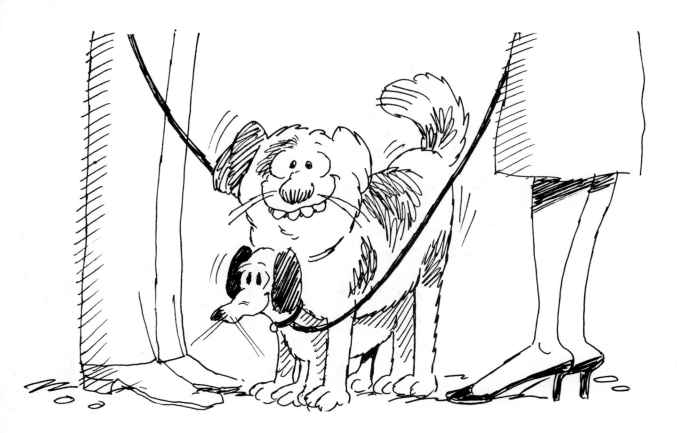

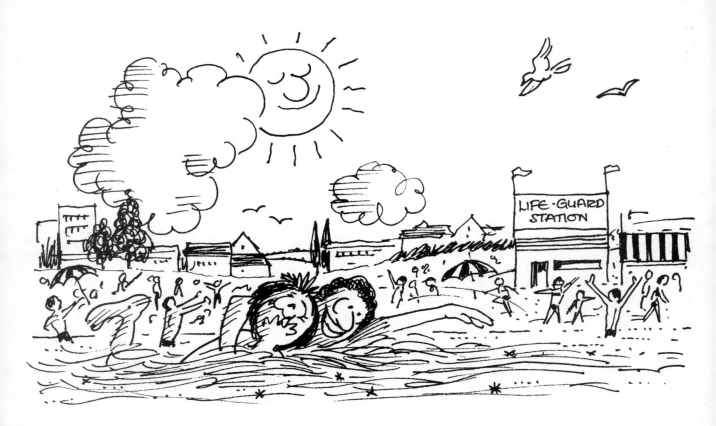

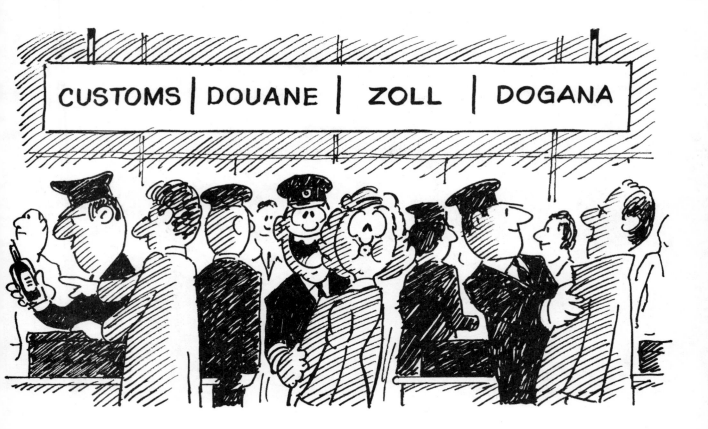

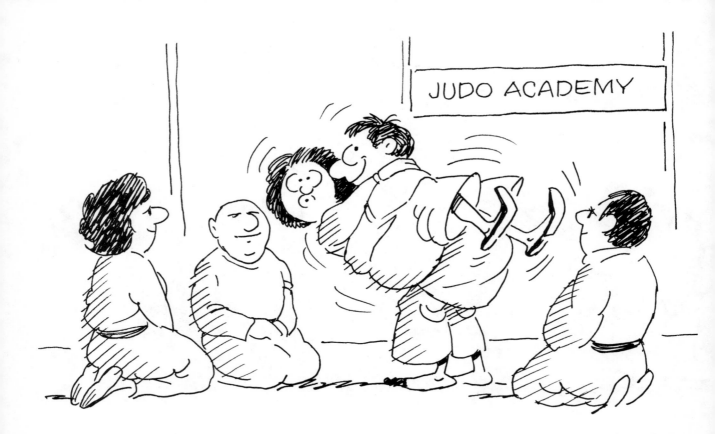

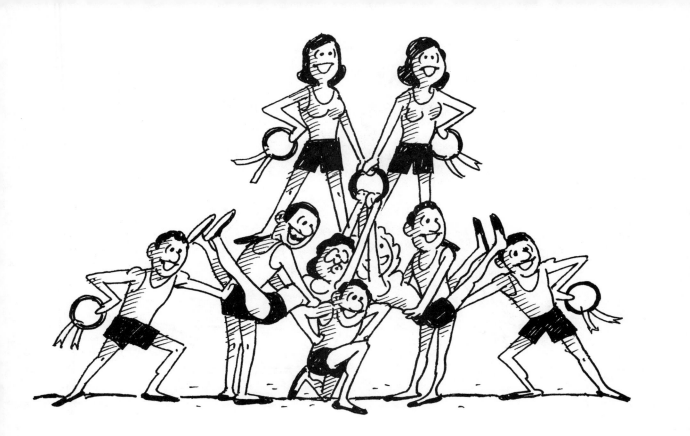

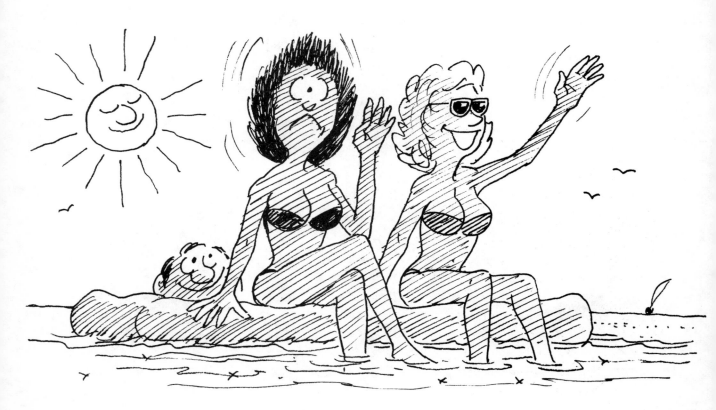

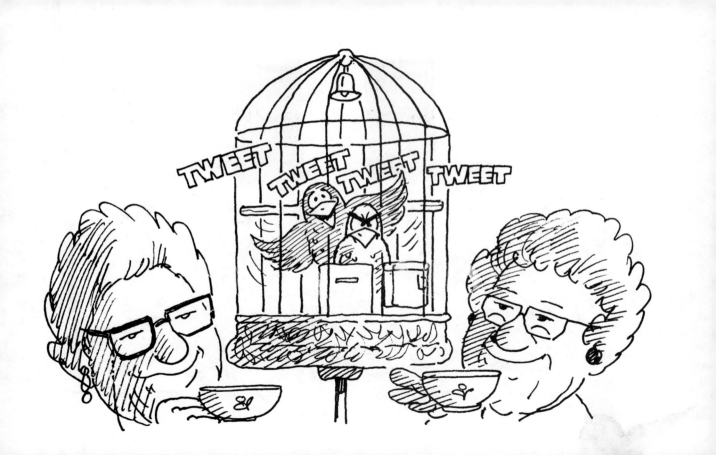

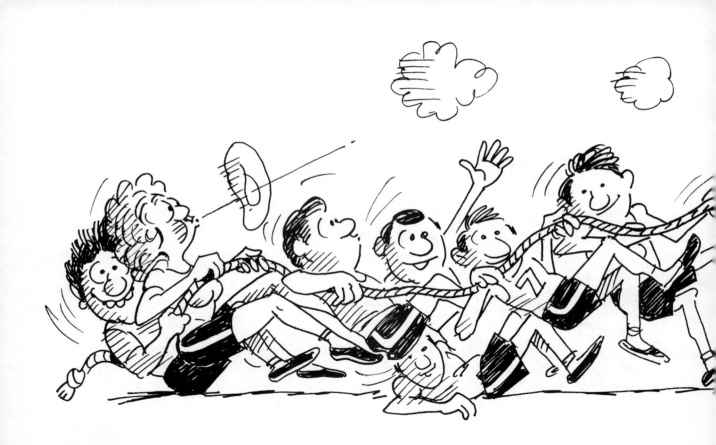

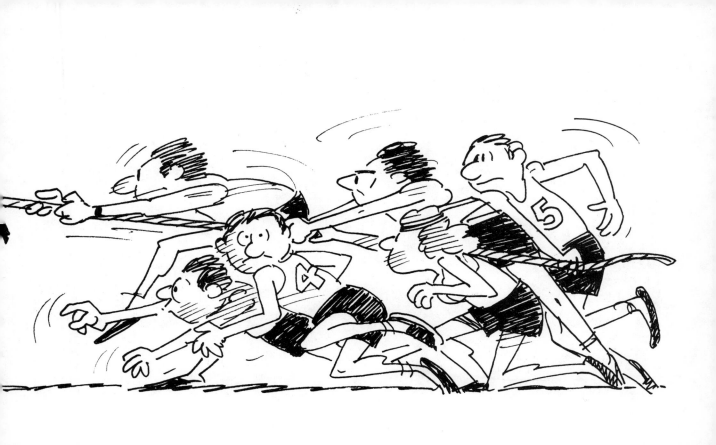

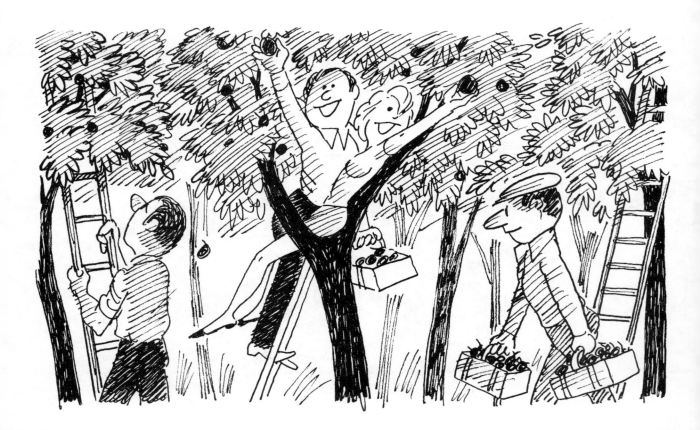

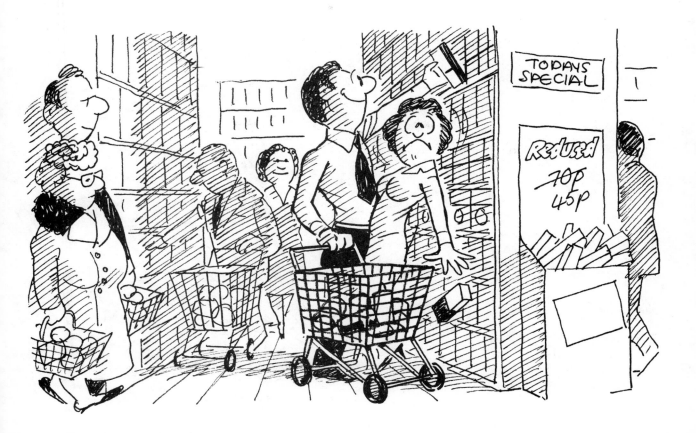

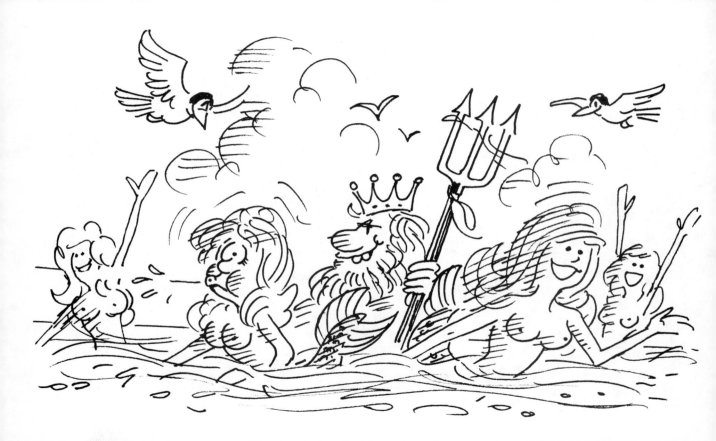

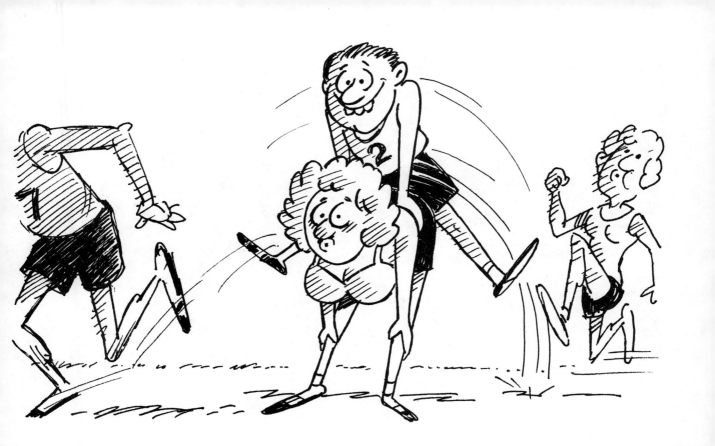

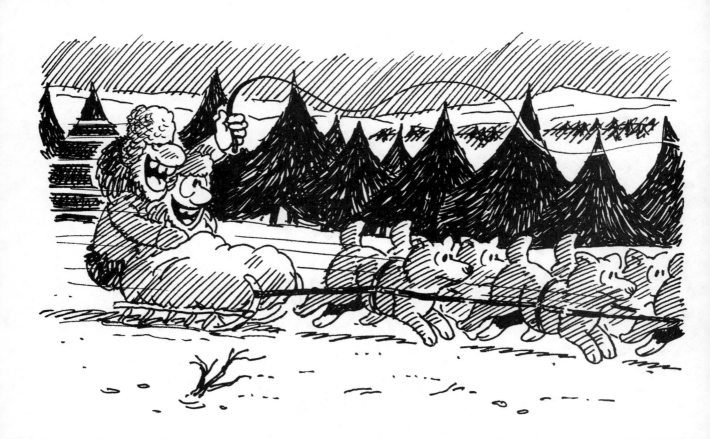

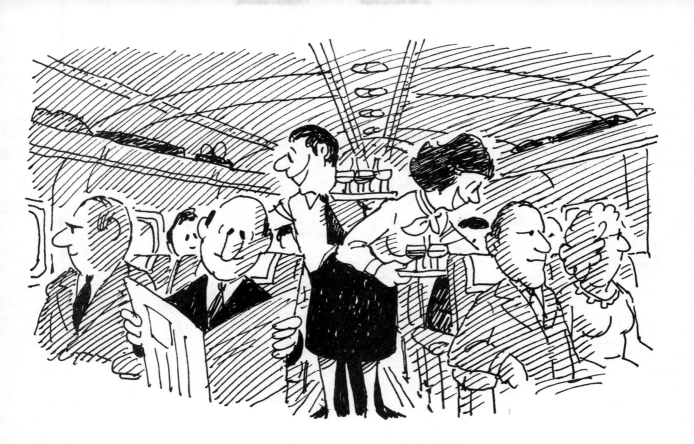

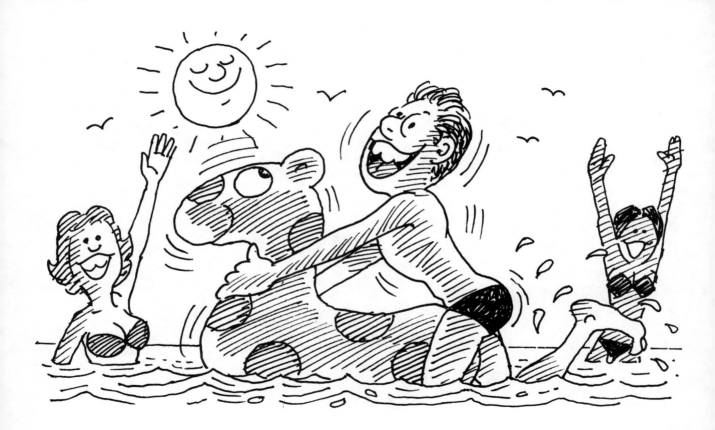

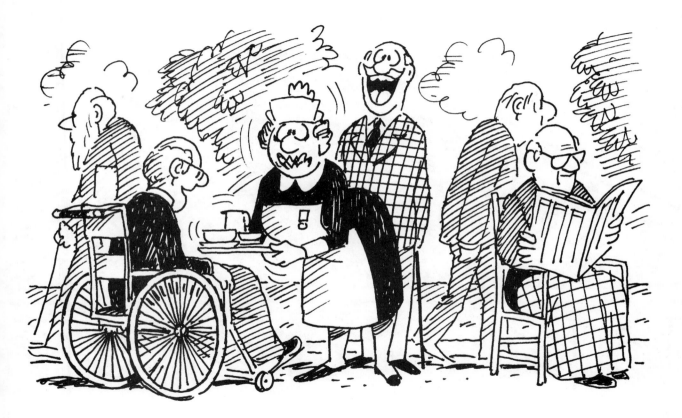

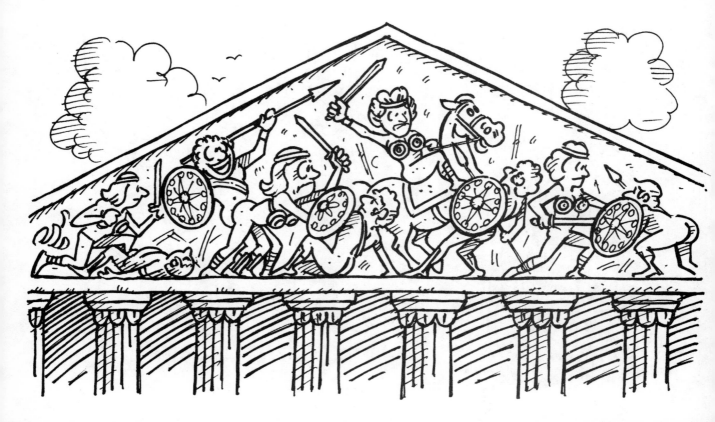

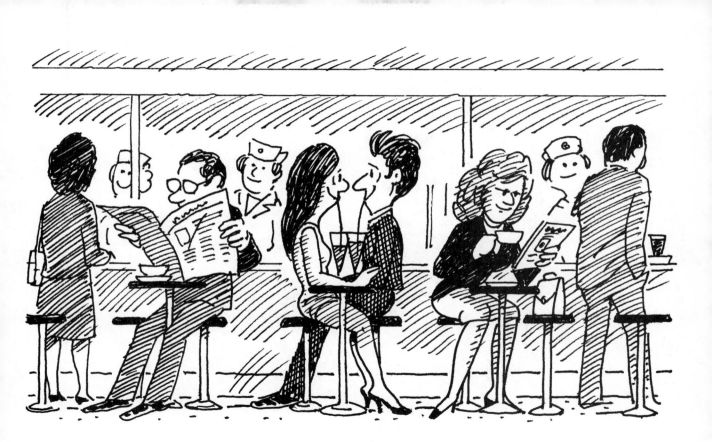

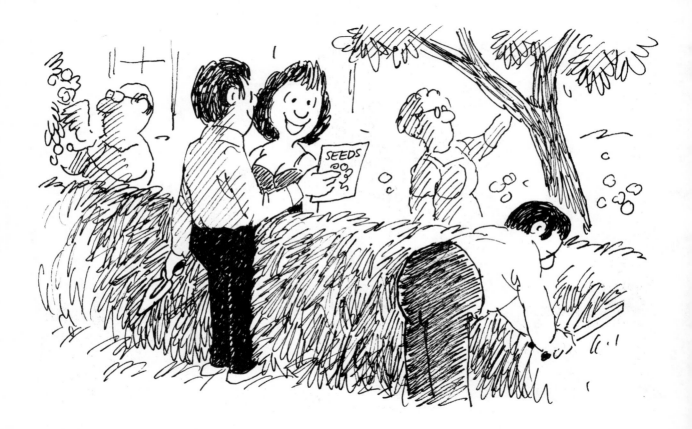

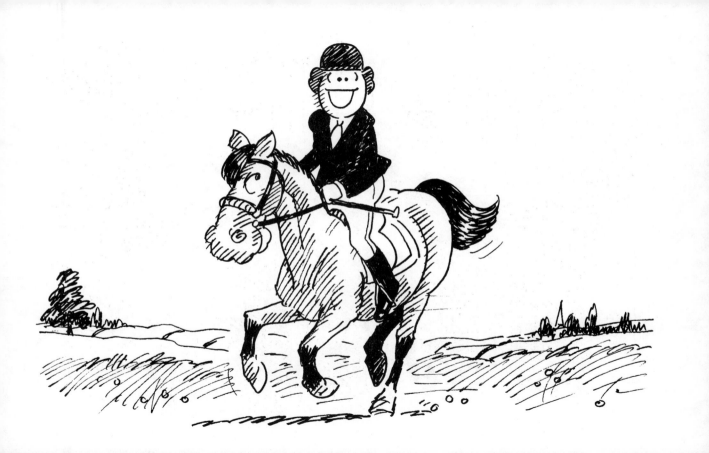

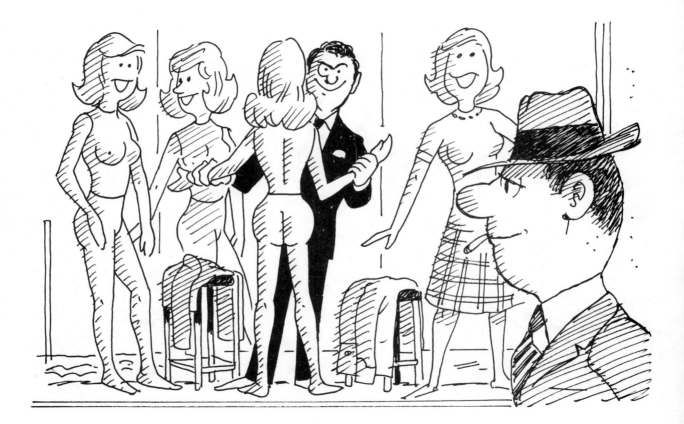

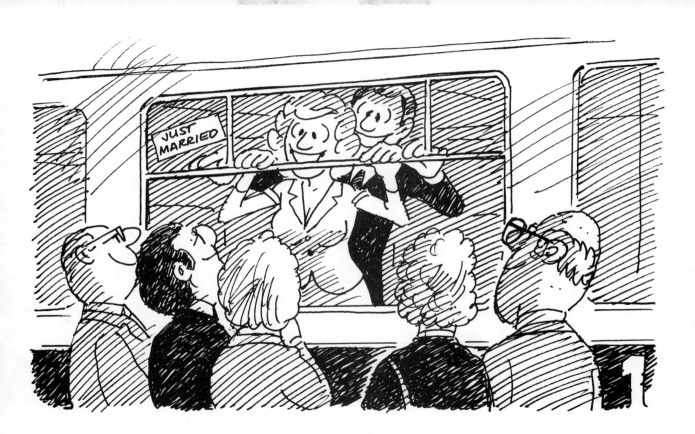

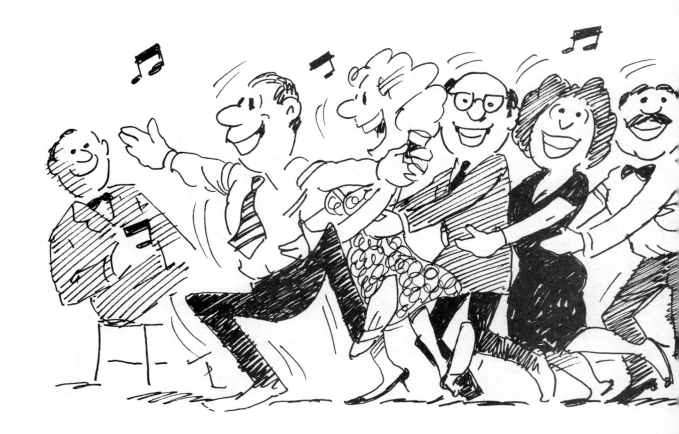

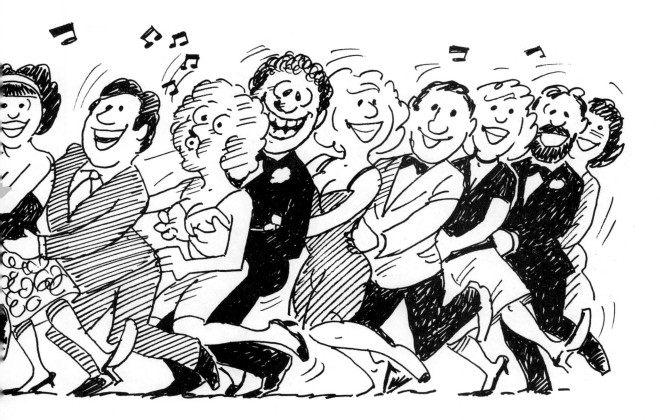

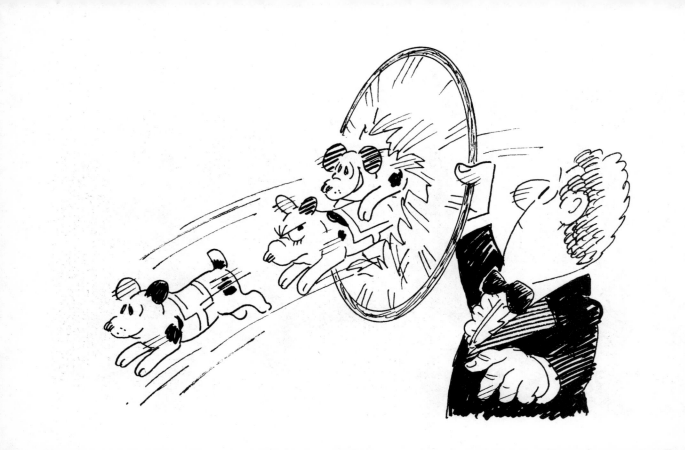

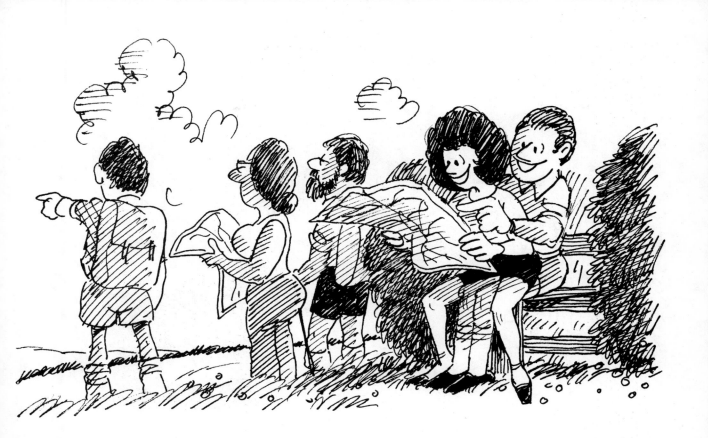

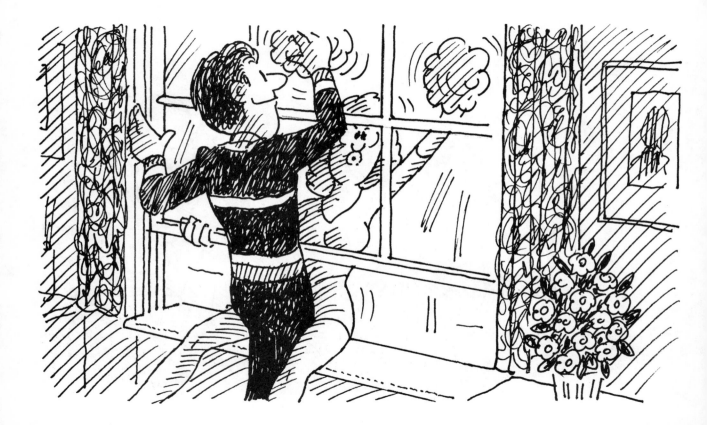

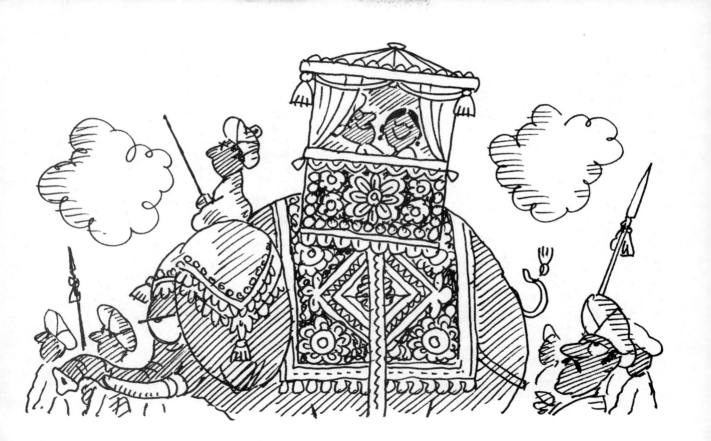

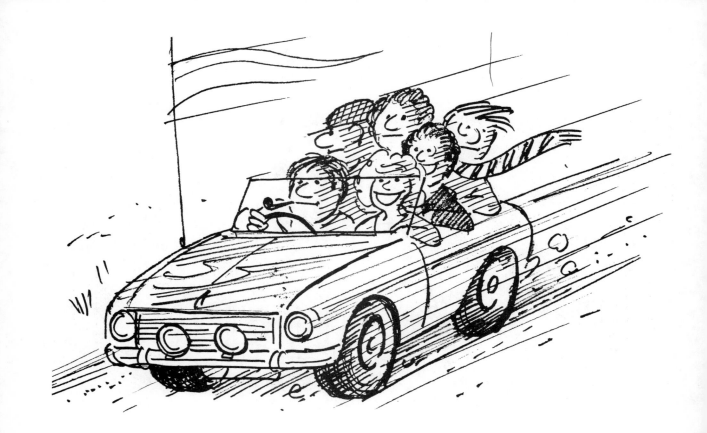

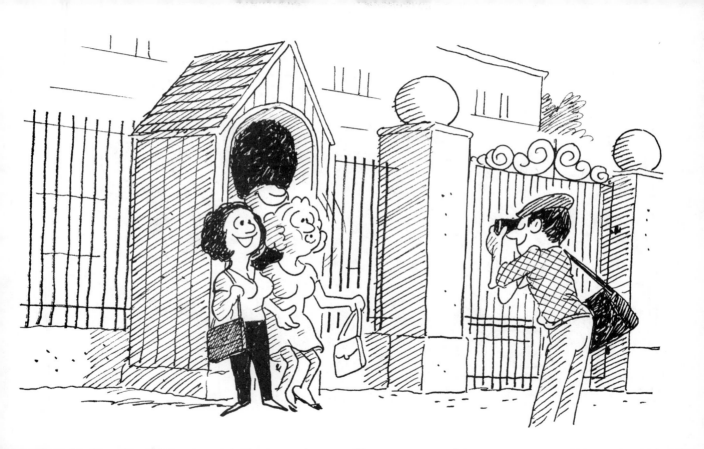

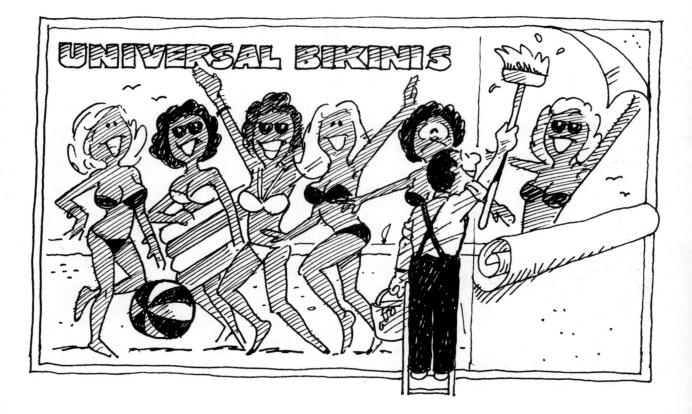

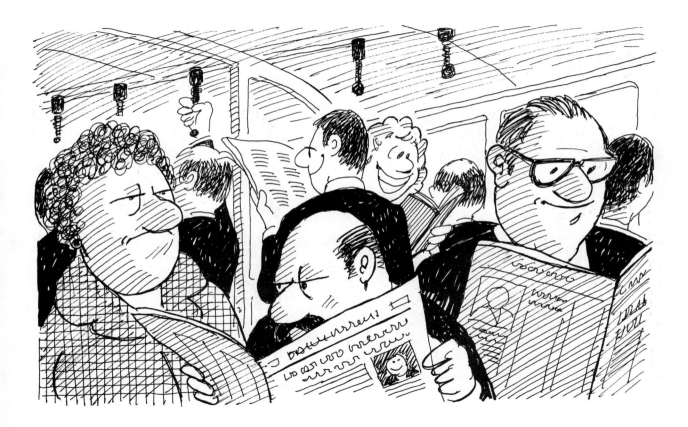

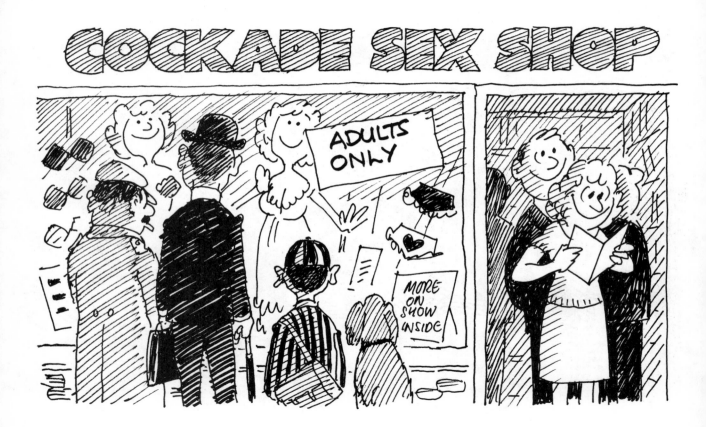

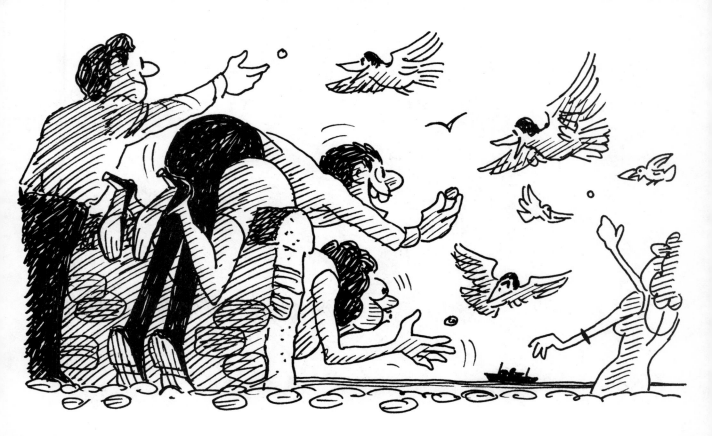

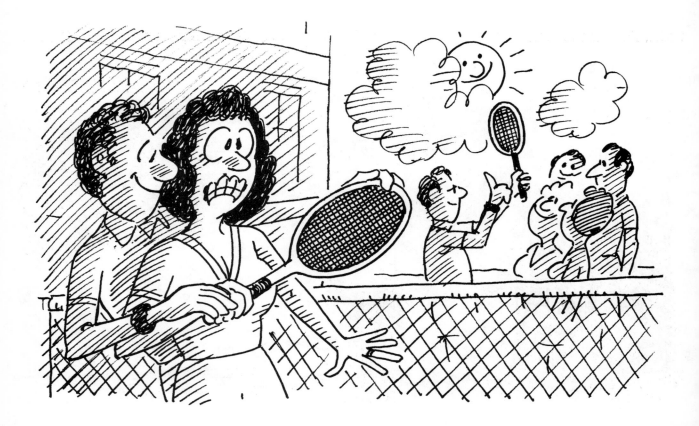

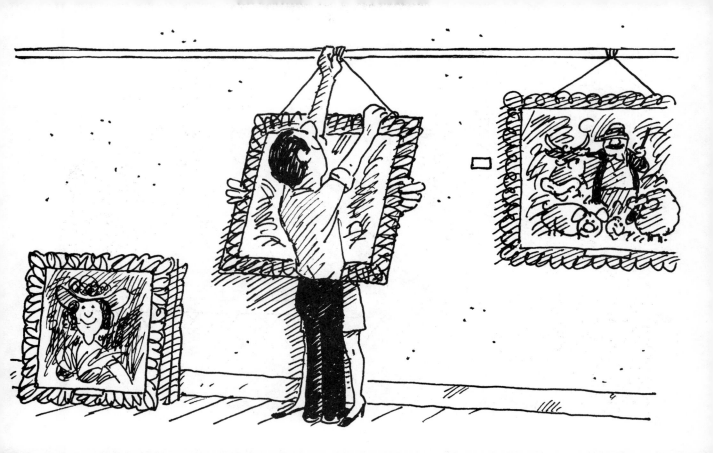

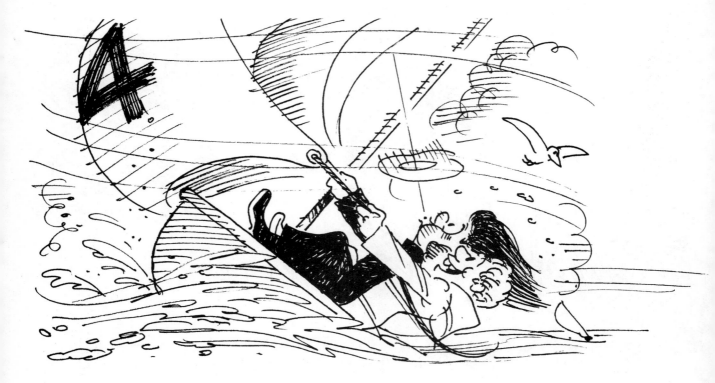

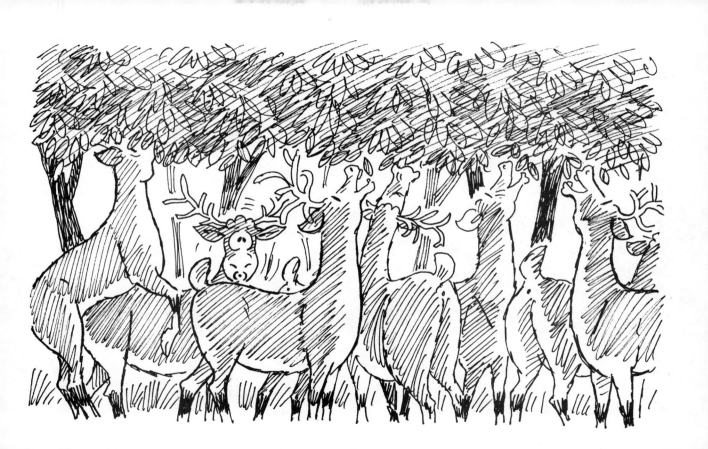

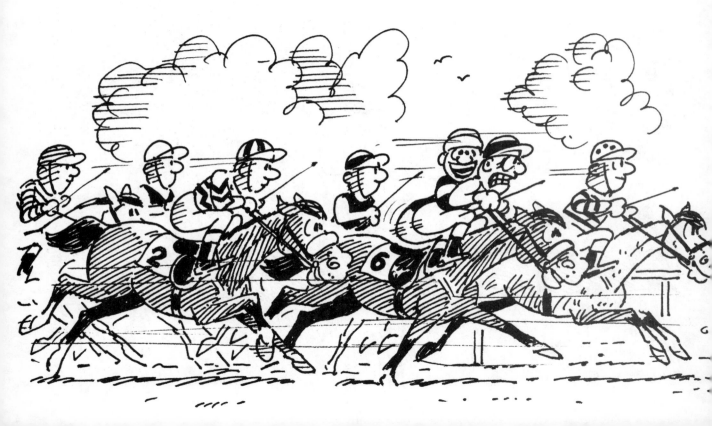

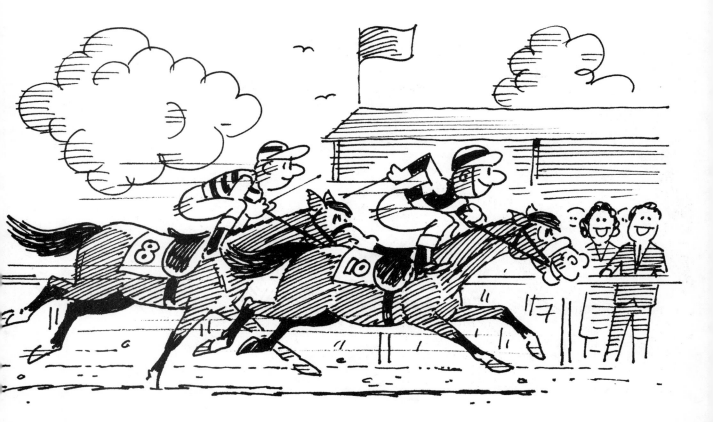

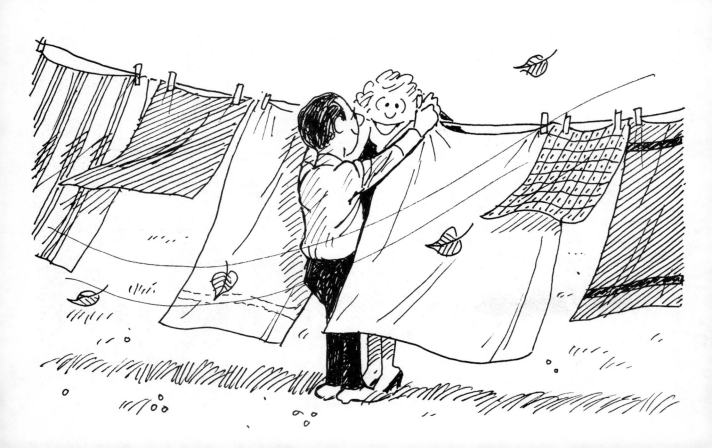

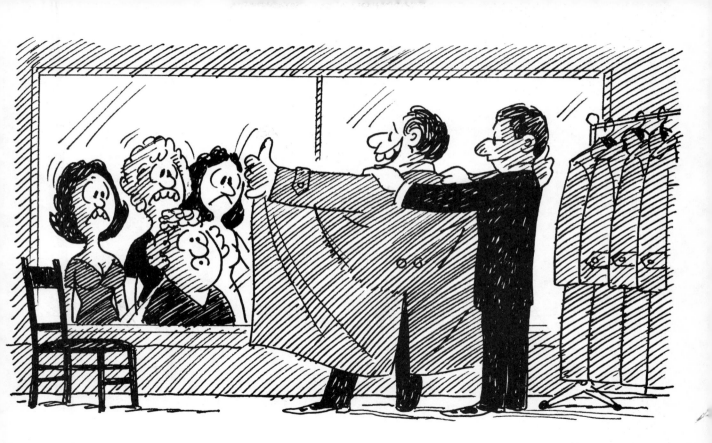

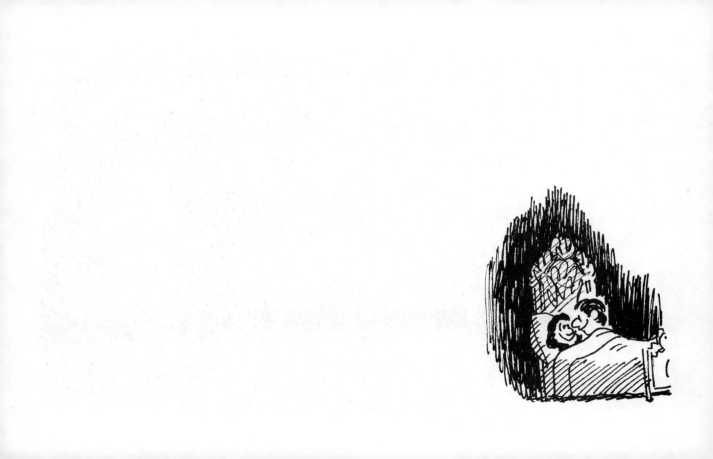

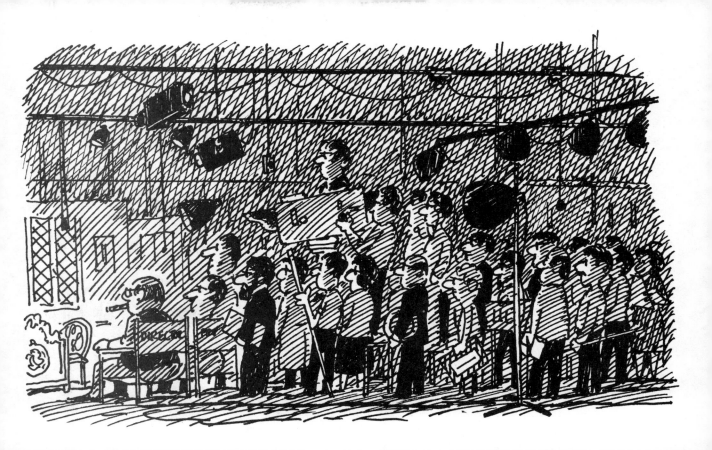

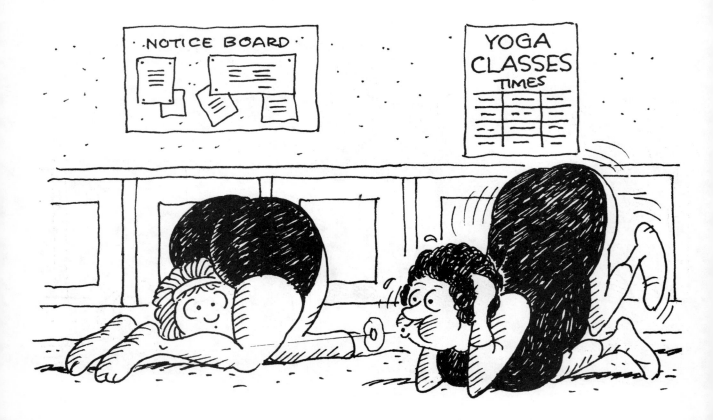

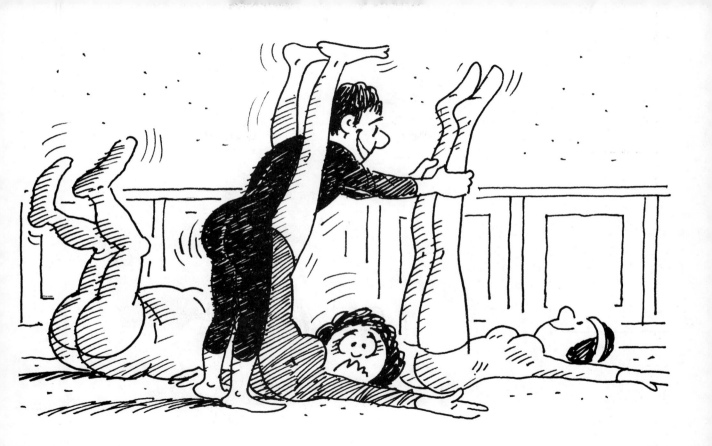

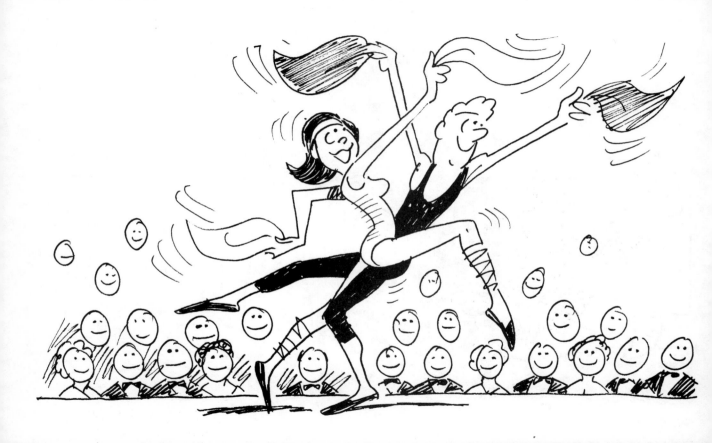

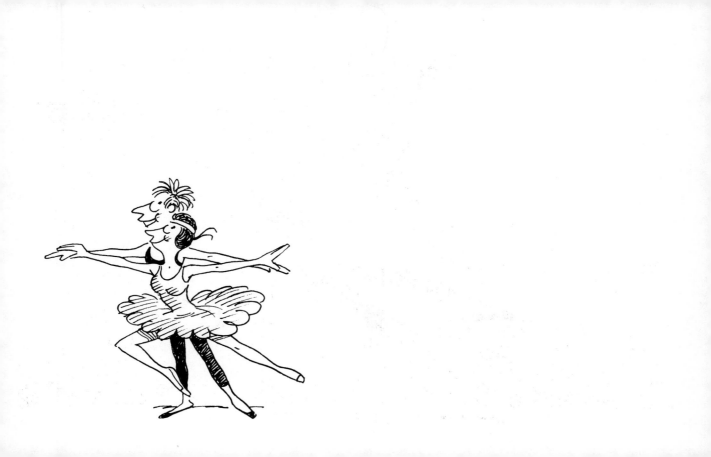